I0840950

Are Yoga & Reiki Healing Evil?

(Rei = ghost) (ki = vapor)

Danny Frigulti

Bible version used:

Scripture is from the King James Version.

Copyright 2018 © Danny Frigulti

Special thanks to Chuck Romer for help on the cover design.

ISBN – 13:978-1727253719

ISBN – 10:172725371X

Other books by the author available at Amazon:

Are Word of Faith Televangelists Misleading Millions?
EXPOSED: The False Faith Healing-Prosperity Gospel
Questions for Word-Faith, Prosperity Believers

Author's website is www.dannyfrigulti.com

Table of Contents

The History of Reiki Healing

Opening Comments

Yoga exercise and Reiki energy healing have become more acceptable around the world and are now openly embraced in the United States of America. This has become of great concern for those who are aware of the historical and spiritual implications of what appears to be a harmless Hindu exercise (Yoga) and a Japanese energy healing therapy (Reiki).

By the end of this book, sufficient knowledge on both of these subjects will clearly give you a thorough and accurate description to what comprises Yoga and Reiki healing. You might be stunned to discover that the "spiritual power source" of these two popular and widely accepted *spiritual* activities is *not* from the Holy Spirit Who did signs, miracles, and wonders through the Lord Jesus Christ and His apostles.

Extensive amounts of detailed information presented on both of these controversial topics will be provided for you from people who endorse Yoga and Reiki. I use *their websites* so that you will have accurate facts from *well-informed* people who have insight on these two hotly-debated topics. It is your choice to accept or reject the "obvious truth" about these two daily worldwide practices.

The information contained in these pages is presented for "truth that leads to true Biblical enlightenment" (Ephesians

1:18-20). We should remember there are streams of *false* enlightenment that are found in the world (2 Corinthians 4:4; 11:13-15). The physically resurrected Jesus (Romans 1:3-4) is the true light Who shines out in the darkness (John 8:12). Follow the true light forever.

In 1 Thessalonians 5:22, Christians are told to "Abstain from all appearance of evil." If you claim to be a Christian and are caught up in any of the unbiblical practices that will be exposed in this book, you need to do the right thing and stop doing them by repenting of your sin. Continue in His Word, and the truth will set you free (John 8:31-32).

If you are *not* a Christian, hopefully the numerous facts will convince to have no involvement with Yoga or Reiki and become a joyful Christian. God is looking for those who will worship *only* Him in spirit and truth (John 4:23-24).

When you have finished this book, please do not let it collect dust. Pass it on to someone who needs this guidance and pray for them.

Note:

At the time of this first printing in 2018, all of the websites used for Yoga and Reiki information could be viewed to confirm quotes and information used. Should you go to these websites, you will find more information than what was cited. If any change or website shut down occurs, you can still find these topics online by typing in the section title of the subject. God bless you for taking time to learn this information.

The Evils of Yoga

Some may be surprised or offended by my descriptive title concerning Yoga because it's common to hear people say, "What's wrong with Yoga. It's only sitting, stretching, and breathing for health improvement; so how can it be evil?" However, there is much more to what Yoga represents than many participants realize. When you have finished learning the details of what comprises Yoga, you may be quite surprised, perhaps stunned to find out how millions (even Christians) are involved with something that looks innocent, but packs an evil foundational history.

Many Christians are involved with Yoga and believe there is nothing wrong with this Hindu exercise. I will present what Yoga teaches *during* physical exercise to show if there is definite proof that Yoga exercise conflicts with Scripture. If there is compatibility between Yoga and Christianity (what Jesus teaches), then we should find obvious Biblical evidence and embrace Yoga exercise. If there is Scripture warning us that Yoga is evil, then Christians must not participate in any form or type of Yoga. To do this would be rebellion, which is a serious sin (1 Samuel 15:23).

If you are *not* a Christian, you still need to consider the spiritual consequences of Yoga participation that will be revealed throughout the following pages. It will be explicitly shown that Yoga introduces and guides participants to more than physical conditioning.

Yoga exercise (even with animals) has become quite popular throughout the United States during the last thirty years. Yoga classes are being taught in businesses, fitness centers, health clubs, hospitals, houses, city parks, beach areas, churches, DVDs at home, and college classes. Pictures of people in the Lotus Yoga "Om" position are also found in public education books and in television commercials.

Sometimes the literature describing Yoga or the person teaching it will say, "Yoga is not a religion, but only a type of exercise." Therefore, according to most proponents of Yoga exercise, it can be incorporated with any religion or faith and not be in conflict with the faith or religion of the participant. But is this the truth or a covered lie?

Could Yoga and its exercise positions be connected, united, or linked in any way to any religion? If it is not yoked or united with any religion, then what is Yoga's connection to Hinduism? Where does Yoga exercise gets its power for the spiritual enlightenment that supposedly awakens the divinity within all people? What is Kundalini power? Could Yoga have a demonic connection? Are the chakras powered by evil power or by the Holy Spirit? Why are prayer hands used in Yoga? Do Yoga mantras have a specific purpose? The origin, beginning history of Yoga, and definitions of the components of Yoga will give us our answers.

Various sources I have read say Yoga has been around for about five thousand years. Some say Yoga began in the Indus Valley in northern India where archeological evidence found in Mohenjoharo seals depicts a figure seated upright in the traditional Yoga pose with legs crossed. Others say Yoga was in existence in India prior to this time. What is important is not how long Yoga has been around but what Yoga represents. Therefore, the definition and purpose of Yoga are needed to determine if Yoga is compatible with Jesus and the Bible.

By definition, Yoga means "union" or "yoked" in Sanskrit, an Indian language (sometimes translated "to bind"). So what is Yoga in union with or yoked with? Does it have a God-endorsed spiritual connection with Judaism or Christianity? Since numerous sources teach that it has been in existence for about five thousand years, we need to ask this question. Are there any reliable Hebrew records of God-ordained Yoga being part of the Hebrew culture prior to or during their Egyptian bondage of about four hundred years, or after Moses led them out of Egypt?

A careful reading of the Torah (the first five books of the Old Testament) will show there is no mention of the LORD endorsing Yoga, the seated Lotus pose that honors the god Shiva, Yoga postures called "asanas," or Yoga's specific breathing exercises called "pranayamas." When Moses led the people out of Egypt, he led them out of physical captivity and away from many forms of idol and demon worship that were common among the pagan nations (Deuteronomy 18:9-12). If Yoga was practiced in Egypt thousands of years ago prior to the Hebrew Exodus from Egypt, then it was left behind as an evil pagan practice because it was not God approved. The LORD has always desired for His people to separate themselves from anything sinful and of the devil (2 Corinthians 6:16-18).

In the New Testament, there is no mention of Yoga used as a way to connect with the true God in prayer, postures (asanas), or special breathing to improve your spiritual and physical health. Spiritual health comes through repentance of sins, and following and obeying Jesus with your heart (Acts 2:38-39). Physical health is a combination of proper diet, sleep, rest, and exercise. Nowhere in the Bible does it encourage people to be in "union" or be "yoked" with Yoga. So if a person decides to practice Yoga, then where or with what does Yoga establish its yoke and union? To know the answer to this, we must expose more about Yoga.

Meaning of the Lotus Position

The seated position of Yoga with legs crossed and wrists on your feet or wrists on your knees has a specific purpose. It is called the Lotus position or pose, and spelled two ways (padmasana or padma-asana). Pictures of Indian gods and goddesses, also known as deities, sitting in this position are common in the Hindu religion. Therefore, what does the Lotus position tell us about Yoga?

…According to Hinduism, within each human is the spirit of the sacred lotus. It represents eternity, purity, divinity, and is widely used as a symbol of life, fertility, ever-renewing youth… In the postures of hatha yoga, the lotus position, *padmasana*, is adopted by those striving to reach the highest level of consciousness, which itself is found in the thousand-petalled lotus chakra at the top of the head. (Lotus magick?). (http://www.lotussculpture.com/my_articles_lotus.htm).

Insight: No Bible verse teaches that "within each human is the spirit of the sacred lotus," which represents "divinity." This teaching about the Yoga Lotus position verifies that Yoga is part of the Hindu religion. So those who say that Yoga is not religious in any way are not telling the truth. Biblical purity does not come from the spirit of a Lotus flower. It comes from repenting of our sins, and receiving Jesus as our Lord and Savior (John 1:12; Romans 10:9-10). When this occurs, we receive the Holy Spirit (Acts 2:38). What purity we have is given to us through God's grace (Ephesians 2:8- 9). Also, the reference to the "lotus chakra at the top of the head" is proof that Hatha Yoga, sometimes said to be *only physical* Yoga, is connected to the spiritual realm where the seven chakras reside and respond to energy forces from the evil spirit realm. This occult energy is known as "Kundalini power." Therefore, the Hatha Yoga poses used are not for physical exercise *only*. They have a spiritual connection which enhances Yoga. So let's learn about "The Lord of Yogins."

Glory of Lord Shiva

Om. I bow with folded hands to Lord Siva, Who is Lord of the universe (Jagat-Pati), world's teacher (Jagad-Guru)…who is full of light (Jyotirmaya)…Who is the Lord of Yogins (Yogeesvara)…Who is the storehouse of knowledge… Hatha Yogins awaken the Kundalini Sakti that is lying dormant in the Muladhara Chakra by Asana, Pranayama, Kumbhaka, Mudra and Banda, take it above through different Chakras (centers of spiritual energy) Svadhishthna, Manipura, Anahata, Visuddha and Ajna and join it with Lord Siva at the Sahasrara, the thousand-petalled lotus at the crown of the head. (Swami Sivanada, page 1).

In Me the universe had its origin. In Me alone the whole subsists…
(http://www.sivanandaonline.org/public_html/?cmd=display section§ion_id=1040).

Insight: The first four lines of this quote describe Lord Siva as one to bow down to (to worship), Lord of the universe, the world's teacher, full of light, and a storehouse of knowledge. The Bible identifies Jesus as King of Kings and Lord of Lords (Revelation 19:16), as Master and Teacher (Matthew 23:8), as the true light (John 1:4-10; 8:12), and has all the treasures of wisdom and knowledge (Colossians 2:2-4). The above quoted description of a Hindu god/deity called "Lord Shiva" or "Lord Siva" is what you are recognizing, accepting, and imitating (seated pose) as a teacher of Yoga, or if you are involved with Yoga. If you are a Christian, you can't mix

Yoga with Jesus, the Son of God, because Yoga imitates the unholy realm of gods. This is against the Holy purity of Biblical teachings. (Exodus 20:3-5).

Also, for those who insist Hatha Yoga is only physical, this information states Hatha Yogins awaken the Kundalini Sakti spiritual energy that lies dormant in the Muladhara Chakra through Asana (Yoga poses), Pranayama (Yoga breathing-inhalation and exhalation techniques), and Mudras. Mudras are prayer hands placed in front of your heart or in front of your forehead that permit you to pray to the god within you as your thumbs point to you, or point to the chakras in you.

The word "Om," at the beginning of this quote, is a sound used when seated to resonate or vibrate one's will to recognize, call out, and connect with the so-called universal omnipresent god. For Christians, there is one Lord and one God (1 Corinthians 8:4-6), and they connect with Him through prayer, praise, and reading the Bible. And no matter what the Hindus or Yogis believe about the origin of the universe, it was not created by Lord Shiva. Jesus and His Father created and spoke all things into existence (Genesis 1; Isaiah 44:24; 45:12; John 1:1-3; Colossians 1:16-17).

It's obvious that the seated Lotus position in Yoga is an "occult doorway" to more evil. It is not a sin to sit with your legs crossed and relax your hands on your legs. But when you form the fingers on your hands to represent the "Om" symbol, then you are specifically appealing to a Hindu god. The progression of evil and sin will be confirmed through more details that take place during Yoga activity in the next section.

Exposing Yoga's Components:

Om, Mantras, Poses,

Breathing, Chakras, Mudras

The last section revealed that Lord Shiva, in his Lotus pose, is Lord of Yoga, so let's begin to expose what Lord Shiva wants his Yoga participants to practice as a lifestyle. This section will reveal various unbiblical and occult activities commonly occurring during Yoga classes. The first component we will define is the word "Om," also spelled "Aum."

The Meaning of Om

Before the beginning, the Brahman (absolute reality) was one and non-dual. It thought, 'I am the only one - - may I become many.' This caused a vibration which eventually became sound, and this sound was Om. Creation itself was set in motion by the vibration of Om.

The vibration produced by chanting Om in the physical universe corresponds to the original vibration that first arose at the time of creation. The sound of Om is also called Pranava, meaning that it sustains life and runs through Prana or breath. (http://www.omsakthi.org/worship/mantra.html).

Insight: This article says that Brahman, a Hindu god, was "before the beginning." Read Colossians 1:16-18. Verse 17 says, "And He (Jesus) is before all things, and by Him all things consist." Life in abundance and eternal life are found in Jesus (John 1:4; 10:10; 1 John 5:11-13), not in Pranava or Prana breath. These Om quotes "vibrate" with deception concerning sound and words. Do all of our words and sounds please the Lord Jesus, or do some please evil spirits?

What Does Ohm Mean in Yoga?

Om or Aum is a mantra that is often chanted at the beginning and end of yoga sessions. Om is both a sound and a symbol rich in religious meaning and depth. It is said to be both the sound of the creation of the universe, and the sound of silence. It represents both the highest level of divinity and the path to enlightenment.... In the Hindu religion Om is considered a sacred sound. Many Hindus consider Om to be the first sound of creation. Hindus also believe that everything in the universe, even inorganic objects, originated in Om and are therefore alive with vibration based on the sound of Om. (http://healthyliving.azcentral.com/meaning-om-yoga-8462.html).

Insight: The word "Om" is called "rich in religious meaning and depth." Therefore, according to Hindu teachings, anyone who hums or chants "Om" is chanting "a sacred sound." Keep in mind that "Om" is taught as the source of all mantras. This means no matter what mantra a person uses in Yoga, (this includes Christians involved with Yoga), that the original source and foundational teaching is from another god and another religion. Jesus never taught any vain repetitious mantras. He taught prayer (Matthew 6:7-13; John 14:13). So to hum or chant the Name of Jesus or anything from the Bible does not put you any closer to Him. It puts you closer to Lord Shiva and Brahman, occult gods, who are enemies against the Lord Jesus and the Holy Spirit. This is sin. Also, true enlightenment comes from Jesus, the true light from heaven (John 1:4, 9; 8:12), because He is the highest of divinity from eternity (John 1:1-3; Colossians 1:16-17).

Note: Some believe that when Yoga participants sit with their legs crossed with palms up, they have the fingers on their hands positioned in a specific way to represent "Om." They touch their thumb to their forefinger to form an "O." To form an "M," they hold the remaining three fingers, curved or straight, away from the "O." This hand pose spells the word "Om" which honors the Hindu god, Brahman.

Mantras

Mantra is a religious or mystical syllable or poem, typically from the Sanskrit language. Mantras are primarily used as spiritual conduits, words or vibrations that inculcate concentration in the devotees. Mantras are also integrated in religious rituals to remove obstacles, avoid danger, reduce foes, or accumulate wealth. Mantras got their origin from the Vedas of India.

The word "Mantra" has been derived from Sanskrit. Mantra contains two words – "man" which means "to think" (also in manas "mind") and suffix "tra" which means "tool," hence a literal translation would be "instrument of thought."… Mantras are energy-based sounds. (Do Mantras attract evil energy?). (http://www.iloveindia.com/spirituality/mantras).

Insight: These "Mantra" facts establish that mantras are religious, mystical, and are spiritual conduits for use in religious rituals. So to say Yoga is not a religion ignores the fact that "Mantras are also integrated in religious rituals" while doing Yoga. And the word "Mantra" means "instrument of thought," which will now be shown as another term for what occultists call "thought forms."

Welcome to the Abode of Gods – Mantra

The word Mantra means "thought form" – the image in our mind. And by giving it a "word" or "words" and reciting it, this "thought form" or "image" becomes "alive." These sacred utterances used in worship are called Mantras…. Here we shall try to restrict to the practice of Mantras and to the followers of the occult. Mantras essentially represent a deity, an image of the cosmic force. This subtle energy gets activated through the recitation of the Mantras. Mantra is a bridge that links the worshippers and the worshipped. Hence mantra is the essential mode of worship and it also becomes the most effective tool for magic. Also listed in this article, concerning the power of Mantras, was their ability to "communicate with spirits," "cure diseases," "acquire supernatural powers," and "worship a deity for exalted communion," or "blissful state. (Mantras aren't Biblical!). (http://www.jagjituppal.com/spiritual-knowledge/24-mantra.html).

Insight: Mantras are sacred utterances used in the worship of deities and are said to be "the most effective tool for magic." Magic power is found in the occult realm where legions of demons move to and fro. Magic is not found in Jesus. And mantra power will also help you "communicate with spirits." What kind of spirits? Would you believe demonic spirits? Certainly not Holy angels, for they are commissioned by the LORD (Psalm 103:20-21). The so-called "subtle energy" is a cover term to hide the fact that this "subtle energy" is evil energy. Several years ago I became friends with a witch who renounced her sin of witchcraft and became a Christian. She explained how easy it was for witches to activate and use thought-forms with specific hand motions to connect with demonic spirits. More exposure on "thought forms" should convince you of the ungodly nature of Mantras.

Thought-Form Magick:
What is a thought-form?

A thought-form is a statue or mental image in the form of your desire. It exists in either the mental or astral plane…. Thought-forms are created through ritual involving intense concentration, repetition, and visualization. In occultism an egrigori is a supernatural intelligence called a thought-form, which is produced by the power of the "will" or visualized by participants in a group... They can be directed toward individuals to protect, or heal, or to harm. Also, thought-forms can be created to perform low level tasks or errands. (http://sacredwicca.jigsy.com/thought-forms).

Insight: Thought-form verbal mantras can be used in Yoga, but are not always used. They have the potential to conjure up egrigoris (evil spirits) that have the ability to heal, harm, protect, or "spirit" around influencing people. Thus, people can summon them mentally or visually and "mantra" out to them. Such entities that respond to one's mental/visual/verbal conjuring already exist in the demonic-astral realm, also called "the fourth dimension." They can respond to those who call on them, according to the chosen mantra-thought form choice. This information is from a Wicca site.

These various sources of Yoga mantra information presented show clearly that there is nothing Holy within any context of mantra speaking, chanting, or humming, and it is occult-based. Mantras can be combined with thought-forms and are for pagans, not for anyone who claims to be a Christian. Prayer is for Christians.

The Purpose of Yoga Poses (asanas)

We now know from previous quoted sources that the union or yoke connection in Yoga is with the Hindu god, Brahman, the universal god consciousness of Yoga. The "Om" union/yoke is not with Jesus. With the spiritual origin and foundation of Yoga established, attention to the meaning and purpose of Yoga poses or postures (asanas) will be explained.

A question that needs to be answered is this; do the physical poses (asanas) have any spiritual connection? The answer is "Yes," because Yoga has its spiritual roots in the Hindu religion. Therefore, anytime you are involved with Yoga for exercise, you are exposed to the Hindu faith.

Certainly "Yoga pose exercise" is not of the Lord Jesus and is not taught in the Bible. Is it possible that some deceived and spiritually influenced people got together thousands of years ago, with spiritual help from evil spirits, to honor or worship demonic deities by physically *and* spiritually (mantras) exercising for the gods?

Caryl Matrisciana produced a DVD in 2007 titled, *Yoga uncoiled from east to west*.[1] It reveals several pieces of information on Yoga from people who know Yoga well. Here are some quotes from the DVD that can be purchased at www.caryltv.com :

1. "Yoga is a Hindu word. Yoga is Hindu discipline to become one with the universal consciousness, which means to become one with god. Which god? Brahma, the Hindu god."
2. "In Hinduism, they have more than 330 million gods."
3. "They believe the serpent power is in every person and the serpent power is sleeping in you."

(This is called Kundalini power, a demonic spiritual force that resides in the occult).

These DVD comments are from Dr. George P. Alexander who also authored a book titled, *Yoga: The Truth Behind The Posture*.

George Alexander was born in Sri Lanka and grew up in India, the birthplace of Hinduism and Yoga. "Many Westerners who practice Yoga today are unaware that the physical positions assumed in Yoga symbolize a spiritual act: worshipping one of the many Hindu gods." Dr. Alexander says: "To a Hindu, Yoga is the outward physical expression of a deep spiritual belief. You cannot separate one from the other." (http://praisemoves.com/about-us/why-a-christian-alternative-to-yoga/).

4. "Yoga is Hinduism." Subhas Tiwari, Professor of Yoga Philosophy and Meditation, University of Arizona. (Yoga DVD).

5. "Hinduism is the soul of Yoga, based as it is on Hindu Scripture and developed by Hindu Sages." (Yoga DVD).

6. "The physical postures of Yoga trigger the supernatural of the god presence." (Yoga DVD).

7. "Every form of the Yoga movement derives from the serpent. When a person practices Yoga, he is actually bowing down to the god of the serpent." Jean Lim, author/speaker, (Yoga DVD).

8. "Can there be a physical Yoga without a spiritual Yoga? The answer is 'no' because they are all part and parcel of the same thing." (Yoga DVD).

These eight quotes from reputable people provide sufficient information proving that Yoga is an important and inseparable spiritual/religious part of Hinduism. Definitely, from ongoing evidence, Yoga is used to make contact with the god Brahman and other gods through the use of poses, and mantras, a type of Hindu prayer. Therefore, Yoga and its mantras are to Hinduism gods as prayer is to the LORD in Christianity. Prayer-mantras used during Yoga have no Bible foundation. The type of prayer Jesus taught (Matthew 6:9-13) is encouraged by the Holy Spirit and goes to the LORD God in heaven in the Name of Jesus (John 14:13-14). To claim to be a Christian and use Yoga mantras *of any kind*, and then pray to the God of the Bible, is a sin and an insult to the Lord Jesus.

Pranayama - its Function in Yoga Breathing

An important part of Yoga is a breathing technique called "pranayama." Not all Yoga sources give exactly the same definition for "pranayama." By basic definition, what is "pranayama?" Some break it down into the words "prana" and "yama." Others break it down into the words "prana" and "ayama." Definitions I've read from different sources for understanding what pranayama represents were: "life force for breath control," "energy breath force," "vital energy breathing force," or "expansion of the life force through breath control."

This information helps us to know that "pranayama" is a type of Yoga breathing emphasizing breath control with some type of energy or life force that is available to participants. That life force (prana) will be exposed in more detail with forthcoming information. The deep and emphatic "in and out breathing" (pranayama) is used in Yoga to lead the person to a meditative state, with the mind clearing itself of all thoughts, which supposedly allows one to connect with the inner higher self (what Yoga calls the divinity, divine light, or god within you) to experience a deeper state of relaxation.

Prana:

Master Choa Kok Sui

Master Choa Kok Sui is the Founder and Originator of the Pranic Healing and Arhatic Yoga System, as well as the internationally acclaimed author of the book, *Miracles Through Pranic Healing* (3rd Edition). Originally published in 1987 as *The Ancient Science and Art of Pranic Healing*, Master Choa conceptualized a far deeper understanding of energy healing, using the readily available source of all life-Prana, called Pranic Energy or Vital Life Force…. A prolific author, other books written by Master Choa Kok Sui include: *Pranic Psychotherapy* (1990), *Advanced Pranic Healing* (1992), *Pranic Crystal Healing* (1996)…. These powerful techniques use ancient technology in original and creative combinations in order to activate and align the chakras and to awaken the Kundalini energy or "the sacred fire." (http://pranichealing.com/master-choa-kok-sui).

Insight: The above quote shows that "prana" is more than the air we breathe around us. To those who believe in Arhatic Yoga or "prana" energy healing, "prana" is a spiritual energy breath force and is readily available to anyone who desires an encounter with this invisible energy. We also find this source teaches the chakra connection with Kundalini energy and calls it "the sacred fire." The "sacred fire" is a common term found in witchcraft. Type in "Wicca, the sacred fire" and you will find sufficient information revealing the demonic verification of "the sacred fire" energy. Satan's demonic influence is worldwide (Ephesians 2:2; 1 John 5:19). And so are his many deceiving energy healing techniques, whether they be Universal healing, Reiki healing, Prana healing, or any type of psychic-occult energy healing power. Scientific healing methods are not from the LORD, because He cannot be put into a human-scientific formula and then be forced to heal by submitting to our will and desire. Before leaving the pranayama/prana section, more insight on "chakras" is needed to warn of the many dangers of Yoga.

Health And Yoga Newsletters

Understanding Pranayama – Pt. II

...Pranayama serves to heat that quantum of Prana which then ascends along the spinal column into the Ajna Chakra.

When sufficient heat is generated within the system, the Ajna Chakra sends a feedback to the base (the mooladhara) of kundalini and the dormant potential energy is awakened to increase the energy flow to the Ajna Chakra. This is the purpose of Pranayama. While Pranayama serves to awaken the kundalini, certain Pranayamas are done to purify the carrying channels so that this increased energy can be handled appropriately. (Christ's blood purifies *all* from sin). (http://www.healthandyoga.com/html/news/pran_underp2.aspx).

Insight: It is obvious that Pranayama is not normal athletic breathing to bring oxygen to the lungs. Its purpose in Yoga is to get the participant to a spiritual state which opens the door for demonic Kundalini energy to activate the body from the lower spine. Historical Yoga teaches that all people have this coiled spiritual energy dormant in the lower spinal area, and it is released through the specific Pranayama taught in Yoga. When released, Kundalini energy rushes up the spinal column quickly making contact with one's mind and finally goes out the top of the head. This evil, surging influence of Kundalini-serpent energy alters the soul of a person. Globally, deceived multitudes are moving toward releasing the evil Kundalini power found in Yoga.

Chakras

According to East Indian philosophy we possess seven major Chakras or psychic centers on the body. Each one of these forms a bridge, link, or energy transformer; changing pure (higher) energy into various forms, and connecting the four bodies (i.e. Spiritual, mental, astral, and physical) together. The chakras are located along the nadies (a network of psychic nerves or channels) and follow the autonomic nervous system along the spinal cord.… Chakras correlate with major acupuncture points along the "governing vessel meridian" (acupuncture term).… Chakras are visible to clairvoyant sight as variously colored rotating circles or funnels. In the East they are described as petaled flowers or lotuses. While in Western Shamanism they are divined as Spirit Tunnels. (Does chakra energy sound anything like the Holy Spirit?). (http://wicca.com/celtic/chakras/chakra.htm).

Insight: Chakra teachings are definitely an integral part of the Yoga components and are also found throughout occult teachings. Remember, the quick, demonic Kundalini serpent power rushes up through the spinal column to reach all seven chakras. This source says the purpose of each chakra link is to be a transformer of energy into various forms to connect the four bodies, and one body is referred to as the "astral body," which is an occult term. We are also told that chakras are visible to clairvoyants. Some clairvoyants have the ability to see into the invisible spiritual realm to see evil spirits, auras, and sometimes inside the human body. The spiritual gift of clairvoyance is not listed in the Bible as a gift from the Holy Spirit but is commonly used among psychic and occult practitioners. The chakras are described as colored rotating circles or funnels, and demonic Shamanism refers to them as "divined spirit tunnels" because spirits travel through these tunnels. In the occult, chakras have also been defined as "gateways to other worlds." This information is devastating proof that there is nothing Holy and God-pleasing about Yoga. For thousands of years, people have been stretching, breathing, and exercising without any Yoga involvement and have lived in good health, so why get involved with evil exercise if you love the Lord Jesus of the Bible?

Mudras and Yoga Prayer (Namaste)
What is a Mudra?

Mudras are described as hand positions…. A Mudra locks and guides energy flow and reflexes to the brain. Together with Bhandas, Mudras redirect the energy flow, linking the individual pranic energy with the universal force. (**Note:** Yoga hand positions are pranic energy guides to deception). (http://www.thesecretsofyoga.com/Mudras/What-is-a-Mudra.html). If you have trouble with this web address, type it in without the http:// and you will find the quoted information.

Insight: Mudras are different hand positions used during Yoga classes, and the purpose is to guide energy flow and response to the brain. The main ones we will focus on are the Mudra that points to one's heart and the Mudra that points to one's head. Earlier information revealed the occult aroma of pranic energy and the "universal force" that counterfeits the

Holy Spirit. Hand positions that direct/guide spiritual energy are not to be treated lightly or ignored.

Why Prayer Hands in Yoga?
Yoga Flavored Life

Anjali Mudra (pronounced UHN-juh-lee muhd-RAAH) is a gesture that is a part of almost all yoga classes. It may be used at the beginning or end of class…. Anjali mudra is also referred to as prayer hands. The palms of the hands are brought together in front of the heart.

By bringing our hands together at our heart center we are connecting to both the right and left sides of the brain. This is symbolic of uniting both our masculine and feminine energies. It is said that the right hand represents the divine self and the left hand represents our worldly nature. The hand gesture of Anjali Mudra is often accompanied by the greeting Namaste which means, "The light in me bows to the light in you." **Note**: Some sources teach that Namaste means, "The divinity/god in me bows to the divinity/god in you." (http://www.yogaflavoredlife.com/philosophy/why-do-we-use-prayer-hands-in-yoga.html).

Insight: The Bible has nothing to say about uniting our masculine and feminine brain energies, because such a teaching is not needed to grow spiritually in Christ. No body part is mentioned in Scripture as representing the divine self. Only the LORD has an eternal divine nature, and He shares it (the Holy Spirit) with us upon our conversion/salvation

(Acts 2:38; Romans 8:11) which allows us to become partakers (2 Peter 1:4). Christians do not bow to the light in one another by using Yoga prayer hands for any reason, but pagans do. We bow to Jesus because Jesus is the true light (John 8:12). We bow to Him as Lord of Lords with hands uplifted in prayer, worshipping, and asking in His Name.

What Does The Term Namaste Mean In Yoga?
Yogic Philosophy

In yoga, namaste means much more than just "I bow to you." Instead, it acts as recognition of mutual respect. According to *The Women's Health Big Book of Yoga,* the term is related to divinity in yoga - namely, the fact that your divinity recognizes the divinity in others. As you make the hand gesture and bow at the end of class you're giving kudos to your instructor and the other students as you recognize each other's divinity. (Have you sinned by saying "Namaste"?). (http://www.livestrong.com/article/390926-what-does-the-term-namaste-mean-in-yoga/).

Insight: This quote shows clearly that Yoga is religious, because it teaches we all have divinity (the nature of God) within us. This divine nature taught in Yoga is acknowledged and received in Yoga sessions around the world daily. When the "Namaste greeting" is given, which recognizes the divinity within each person, it verifies Yoga is religious. The "Namaste greeting" is a clear insult to Jesus Christ and His redemptive work on the cross to forgive our sins. We must be born-again (John 3:1-8) to become partakers of the divine nature (2 Peter 1:4) which indwells us (Romans 8:9-11).

Meaning and Interpretation of Namaste

Because of its global usage, Namaste has many interpretations. In general, the word tends to be defined as some derivation of, "The divine in me bows to the divine in you." This spiritual connection comes from its Indian roots. (http://healing.about.com/od/cultures/a/namaste.htm).

Insight: From earlier sources, we learned Yoga meant being yoked or in union with Brahman, a Hindu god. Again we find that when we say "Namaste," we are referring to "The divine nature within one another," which teaches we are all children of divinity or children of God. Therefore, Yoga teaches we are all children of the divinity Brahman, a Hindu god, also known as a false god among Jews and Christians. Are you realizing how evil the heart of Yoga is, and how it is an enemy of and against the Holy Spirit Jesus gives to those who call Him their Lord and their Savior?

Yoga Asanas and Prayers

It isn't too hard to connect yoga asanas and prayers to each other. Yoga has always been about more than just the physical body; it is descended from a tradition of Hindu religious beliefs. (To Hindus, asanas connect with prayers). (http://yoga.lovetoknow.com/Yoga_Asanas_and_Prayers).

Insight: The spiritual and physical Yoga connection is obvious from this quote. Yoga is definitely a combination of the spiritual and physical realms. The fact that prayer hands are a part of Yoga verifies that Yoga is more than physical exercise. If there is no spiritual intent and Yoga is not religious as some teach, then why have prayer hands (mudras) pointing to the heart and mind (third eye chakra)? Since Kundalini is spiritual energy and Yoga breathing (pranayama) and Yoga positions (asanas) are used to activate the serpent Kundalini energy, then truth and reality label Yoga as both religious and spiritual. Yoga is not just physical exercise! Yoga information confirms that Yoga prayer hands are a heart and mind chakra offering to the Hindu gods, exactly what Satan would want for ongoing deception in as many lives as possible. Give your heart and mind to the LORD (Mark 12:30).

Meditation and the Altered State of Consciousness

In Yoga, meditation can be used to focus on your mantra or to empty/clear your mind of any thoughts as you do asanas and pranayama. The teachings or options vary from class to class. The constant pranayama (holding your breath for a few seconds, along with heavy in and out breathing) that can deprive the brain of needed oxygen, combined with meditation that clears/empties the mind, can lead the participant to the altered state of consciousness, which is a

Yoga goal. This makes the mind vulnerable to "thought input" from evil spirits and enhances the possibility of the Kundalini serpent power rushing up through the spine.

However, Yoga students are sometimes taught that these thoughts are from the higher self or "supposed divinity" within all people. Once Yoga followers achieve this Kundalini surge, they believe they have attained a higher god-consciousness. If you are a Christian, please remember that Yoga meditation and pranayama have nothing to do with meditating on God's Word. Psalm 1:1-3 teaches meditation.

When meditating on Bible verses, Christians start by confessing any sin active in their life, including sinful thoughts. With a clean and pure heart before the LORD, the focus is on verses we believe God wants for our spiritual growth and for strengthening our foundation in Jesus. And we do not engage in any special breathing to clear our mind to receive more insight from Him. Confessing our sin, if needed, is sufficient to clear the mind to pray, read, and helps us memorize Scriptures. No type of "mantra" repetition of verses is to be used (Matthew 6:7).

Please remember, breathing techniques do not get you closer to Jesus, regardless of *how you feel* during your Yoga exercise. It just might be an evil spirit you are "feeling" around you because of your anti-Christian exercise. Still, some Christians who teach Yoga believe that as you breathe in you can "breathe in the Holy Spirit and breathe out anything that is not from God." There is no Scripture teaching us we can inhale/breathe in the Holy Spirit when exercising. And we don't breathe out what is not from God. We confess our sins, and He forgives us (1 John 1:7-10). If you are a Christian, you have the Holy Spirit in you (Romans 8:9-11; 1 Corinthians 6:19). No one can inhale or force in the presence of God's Spirit through exercise and breathing.

From what has been presented about Yoga, it is clear that Yoga has become an ever-growing launching platform for occult principles, such as mantras, mudras, chakras, and Kundalini spiritual power. And the desire to pursue Yoga, despite the evident occult connection, doesn't seem to be turning away the multitudes who just want to feel good when doing Yoga. Apparently, many do not care if pranayama breathing, mantras, and evil poses (asanas), which mimic gods, make them feel good. Deceived, some are content to reap the physical benefits of occult exercise and choose to disregard the eventual spiritual consequences of the sin they are sowing (Numbers 32:23; Galatians 6:7-8).

Yoga in America Study 2012

This study shows the magnitude of Yoga's influence and acceptance in America is increasing. These statistics below are frightening because of what we know about the evil components of Yoga:

A 2012 "Yoga in America Study" released by *Yoga Journal* (yogajournal.com) shows that 20.4 million Americans practice yoga, compared to

15.8 million from the previous 2008 study, an increase of 29 percent. The increase in Yoga exercise shows its popularity and the desire for Americans to exercise together. Christians must remember to exercise in ways that are not sinful and offensive to the LORD (Colossians 3:17).

In addition, "practitioners spend $10.3 billion a year on Yoga classes and products, including equipment, clothing, vacations, and media. The previous estimate from 2008 was $5.7 billion."[2] This information shows how people, including Christians, will spend vast amounts of money to participate in sin.

On April 23rd, 2018, the Visalia Times-Delta/Tulare-Advance Register ran a Yoga article on page 3B (Choices) citing a survey conducted by *Yoga Alliance* and *Yoga Journal*. This survey said "the number of Americans doing Yoga has grown by over 50% in the last four years to more than 36 million as of 2016, up from 20.4 million in 2012." In ignorance, Yoga participation continues to grow.

Despite the evil Yoga facts that have been presented, some Yoga instructors claim to be Christians and say, "You can do Christian Yoga." There are online Yoga ministries saying they are Christian, yet they mix Jesus and Scripture with Yoga and its evils. This belief, which promotes so-called "Christian Yoga," will be tested in the next section according to Scripture by reviewing some main components of Yoga with the Bible. Then we will see if the spiritual growth in Yoga glorifies the spiritual growth in Jesus. By definition, a Christian is one who has repented of their sins through placing faith in Jesus' shed blood, death on the cross, and believes He was raised physically from the dead. Then the believer follows Christ and His Bible teachings. We will now see if *any* of Christ's teachings advocate Yoga.

Reasons Why Christians Should not Participate in Yoga:

1. Yoga means "yoked" or "union" with something or someone. That someone is Brahman, a Hindu god. You cannot use the word "Yoga" and say "Let's do Christian Yoga," because by *original definition* Yoga honors and connects you with a Hindu god named Brahman, *not* the Lord Jesus. Also, Shiva is known as the Lord of Yoga. True Christians honor only Jesus as Lord (Revelation 17:14). There are to be no other gods in our relationship with Jesus. Yoga is a pagan teaching. Christians don't need to refine or incorporate pagan physical or spiritual teachings to have a better relationship with Jesus.

2. Mantras (chanting) are meaningless/vain repetitions. Jesus warned about this in Matthew 6:7. Mantras can also be heard by demons in the spiritual realm. This opens the door to possibly inviting demons into the Yoga class, or directly to individuals.

3. No Bible verse teaches that Hindu poses (asanas) will improve your spiritual relationship with Jesus, especially when a pose recognizes "a god." God is looking for those who will worship Him in spirit and truth (John 4:24), not like a Yoga puppet.

4. Jesus never taught His disciples to get into heavy breathing (pranayama) to connect with Him or His Father. He said prayer was enough (Matthew 6:9-15; John 14:13-14).

5. Prayer hands (mudras) that point with thumbs to one's heart or forehead were not taught by Jesus or His apostles. The Bible speaks of praying with uplifted hands or hands spread up toward heaven in 1 Kings 8:22, 54; 2 Chronicles 6:13, and 1 Timothy 2:8.

6. Chakra importance was never taught by Jesus and you can't find the word "chakra" in the New Testament in reference to the Holy Spirit gifts. Also, the Lord Jesus did not say anything good about the serpent/devil (John 8:44) or endorse the wicked serpent Kundalini energy. Jesus conquered Satan, also known as the serpent (Revelation 20:2-3) and his demons through His victory at the cross (Colossians 2:14-15) and His physical resurrection (Romans 1:3-4).

7. God does not want us to empty our mind of anything but sins that need to be confessed so they can be forgiven. An altered state of consciousness to empty

the mind completely is not desired by God. His desire is for us to have a mind that is clearly set on things above (Colossians 3:1-2) and to focus on what is found in Philippians 4:4-8. Then we can grow in the grace and knowledge of the Lord Jesus. Therefore, we abstain from Yoga mantras, mudras, pranayama, and serve Jesus as taught in the Bible.

8. If Jesus walked into a Yoga class, do you think He would join in the activities and sit in the Lotus position to honor a god called lord Shiva? Would He hold His hands displaying the "Om" symbol to honor Brahman, the universal energy god? Would He then begin to chant a prayer verse, imitating a mantra? Would He greet the instructor with "Namaste" (the god in me bows to the god in you)? Would He point prayer hands toward His heart or head to acknowledge the chakra system empowered by serpent Kundalini energy, thus honoring the serpent Satan? Would He do "pranayama breathing" to empty His mind to feel the burning Kundalini energy rush up through his spinal column to achieve divine enlightenment and recognize His full divinity? The answer to these questions is an eternal "NO!" If you are a Christian, prove it by following Jesus and have nothing to do with Yoga (2 Corinthians 6:14-18).

This list of eight reasons shows Yoga exercise is not from the LORD, so why be involved with it? You can teach or participate in exercise classes that will promote good and acceptable health in the sight of the Lord without any trace of Yoga influence. Churches can have exercise classes without using the name of Yoga. Just call it a Christian exercise class that includes various Bible verses and appropriate Christian music. Your exercise music should not sound like you are at a demonic rock concert. Pick praise music that will bless your spirit with both peace and energy that honor Jesus. Then your body can exercise and stretch with comfort as you present yourself completely as a holy and living sacrifice to God (Romans 12:1). This will make Jesus happy.

You don't need to sit in the Shiva honoring Lotus position, do a mudra for chakra recognition, progress to asanas and pranayama, and activate the serpent Kundalini energy to be healthy. Proper stretching with proper breathing and a balanced diet with needed rest will enhance your health.

The spiritual growth in Yoga that eventually leads to the serpent Kundalini awakening has nothing in common with spiritual growth in Jesus that provides forgiveness of sins, leads one to heaven, and bears good fruit (Galatians 5:22-23). Yoga classes are a waste of time (Ephesians 5:15-17). Don't ever think you can wear a shirt with a cross on it, combine Bible reading and Christian music with Yoga exercise, and then it automatically becomes "Christian Yoga" that pleases Jesus. That makes about as much sense as a witch wearing a cross while she's doing a ritual and saying, "I'm doing Christian witchcraft."

All of Yoga's components, whether spiritual or physical, have nothing to do with helping your spiritual growth as a Christian to follow Jesus. Yoga does nothing to cleanse your sins. Every time you do Yoga, you honor the definition of its name and pagan origin which is a sin. And you get deeper into sin by using its evil components (mantras, mudras, pranayama) for exercise. Yoga emphasizes the religion of Namaste, which declares man is God. Jesus said there is only one true God (John 17:3), and He is *not* found in Yoga.

In Christianity, the focus is on Jesus (Hebrews 12:2). When we recognize our sin and admit we need Jesus to forgive our sins (Acts 4:12), then we have the Holy Spirit come into us. According to the Bible, prior to receiving Jesus as Lord and Savior, we do not have any trace of divinity in us. Upon accepting Christ's forgiveness for all our sins, the Holy Spirit comes into us as a gift from God (Acts 2:38) and dwells within us (Romans 8:9, 11). Whatever we do is to be done for the glory of God (1 Corinthians 10:31). Yoga's Lotus position, Om, prayer hands, Namaste greeting, and mantras are done for the glory of lord Shiva and Brahman, not Jesus.

Pastors and elders, do not allow your church to be a welcome sanctuary for the evils of Yoga or you will be guilty of endorsing the evils of Yoga. The Bible and the Lord Jesus do not endorse any of the Yoga components that were presented from *their* websites. Jesus set you free from sin (John 8:31-32), and Yoga's roots, branches, and fruit are sin.

Steps to Freedom From Yoga:

Whether you are a Christian or not, are you still going to say Yoga is okay, ignore God's Word (the Bible), and reject Jesus as the Truth? (John 14:6). If you have been or are involved with Yoga and want to honor God by getting out of it, you must do the following:

1. Confess it as sin to God. Ask His forgiveness and for Him to remove any demonic influence that came into your life because of Yoga. If you *are not* a Christian, admit you have sinned and are repentant (truly sorry) for all your sins. Ask Jesus to come into your life (John 1:12) as your Lord and Savior (Romans 10:9-10). You must believe He died on the cross (1 Corinthians 15:1-6), shed His blood to forgive your sins (1 John 1:7-10), and was raised from the dead as proof that He is the Son of God (Romans 1:3-4).

2. Destroy **all** your Yoga items such as books, pamphlets, Yoga music, emblems, symbols, or anything with a Yoga symbol on it (Deuteronomy 7:25-26; Acts 19:18-19). Do not give these items away that were used for evil.

3. If you have a mat you used and it does not have a Yoga symbol on it, dedicate it to the LORD for future use and put Scripture or a Christian symbol (cross or *ichthus*-fish) on it. Try to memorize Romans 12:1-2, 1 Corinthians 6:19-20, and Colossians 3:17.

4. Do not attend any Yoga sessions again, just to be with old friends for some chit chat and exercise. You left an evil activity, so don't go back to it or get involved with "Transcendental Mantra Meditation" for any reason (1 Thessalonians 5:22).

5. Don't forget that the name "Yoga" means "union" or "yoked" in Sanskrit, an Indian language, and is sometimes translated "to bind." To attach the name "Yoga" to an exercise class and call it "Christian Yoga" is mixing Hinduism with Christianity. Truth mixed with error equals sin. The "word of Yoga" does not glorify the Word of God (John 1:1-3).

Find a good Bible teaching church that does not endorse Yoga. Read your Bible daily and pray often (Philippians 4:6-7). Develop a strong and consistent personal relationship with the Lord Jesus (Acts 2:42-47). Also, get involved with a weekly Bible study. And to complement your overall health, continue exercising, getting proper rest, and eating in a way that pleases the LORD.

Resources used for Yoga information:

1. Matrisciana, Caryl. *Yoga uncoiled from east to west* (DVD), (Menifee, California: Caryl Productions, 2007).

2. Lawson, Chris. *YOGA AND CHRISTIANITY ARE THEY COMPATIBLE?* (Eureka, Montana: Lighthouse Trails Publishing, 2013) p. 3.

3. The Bible.

The Spirit of the LORD is upon Me, because He hath anointed Me to preach the Gospel to the poor; He hath sent Me to heal the broken-hearted, to preach deliverance to the captives, and recovering of sight to the blind, to set at liberty them that are bruised (Luke 4:18).

How God anointed Jesus of Nazareth with the Holy Spirit and with power: Who went about doing good and healing all that were oppressed of the devil: for God was with Him (Acts 10:38).

The History of Reiki Healing

Reiki (pronounced ray-key) healing has become popular and is being promoted in magazines, conferences, hospitals, all-purpose therapy, small gatherings, and on television. People say it helps with physical healings, surgeries, rehabilitation, and eliminates various physical and emotional problems. Reiki healing is also offered by some chiropractors and physical therapists (sometimes it's called "energy therapy," "therapeutic touch," or "Radiance Technique"). It is being used in hospitals across the United States and is very popular in Europe and thrives in Japan, its modern birthplace.

Some advocates of Reiki healing say the power is "universal healing energy" or "universal life energy." They believe this healing energy is around our world and is available for anyone who wants to be a Reiki healer or be healed. Other people disagree with this definition of the power source of Reiki and believe Reiki power is an occult energy power supported by evil spirits.

So what is the "healing source" of Reiki that supposedly produces amazing supernatural results and is captivating many around the world? Is Reiki power the same as the Holy Spirit power Jesus said would come at Pentecost (Acts 1:8)? Or is Reiki power another type of power, perhaps an evil power, which is not from Almighty God and the Lord Jesus Christ? If so, then Reiki healing would be an enemy against God's Holy Spirit Who came from heaven at Pentecost to fill and empower Christ's disciples to preach Jesus (Acts 2:1-47).

To get an understanding of how Reiki energy healing has become quite popular around the world, some history about a man named Usui Sensei, also known as Mikao Usui Sensei, is needed. Dr. Usui is considered to be the modern founder of Reiki.

Who was Mikao Usui?

Mikao Usui "was born on August 15, 1865, in the Japanese province of Gifu, married Sadako Suzuki, and had two children. On March 9, 1926, he died in Fukuyama as a result of cerebral apoplexy."[1] Contrary to what has been written and taught by some, "Dr. Usui wasn't a Christian."[2] Mikao Usui "was a Buddhist."[3] (Tendai Buddhism). After Dr. Usui died, the practice of Usui Reiki "was first brought to the west in 1938."[4]

Mikao Usui believed in what he called *The Five Reiki Principles* that were to be followed daily. They are:

1. Don't get angry
2. Don't worry
3. Show appreciation
4. Work hard (on yourself)
5. Be kind to others [5]

Though these five Reiki principles are guides to self-improvement, they do not emphasize following the true God of creation and conforming to the image of Jesus Christ (Romans 8:29), nor is prayer encouraged. Reiki advocates believe that "Reiki is a method of self-realization, a path to the light, to God, or to oneself."[6] This quote proves Reiki advocates do not believe Jesus is the way and path to Almighty God (John 8:12; 14:6). Reiki supposedly is "built upon the spiritual power of the universe."[7]

Reiki healing also teaches that "All beings into whom life has been breathed have received as a gift the spiritual ability to heal. The same applies to plants, animals, fish, and insects."[8] This teaching directly opposes what is taught in the Genesis creation account. The LORD of creation breathed life into man (Genesis 2:7), and the animals and fish have the breath of life in them (Genesis 6:17; 7:14-15), but plants do not. Also, the Bible teaches that *humanity alone* is given the ability to heal by God's will (1 Corinthians 12:9, 11). Plants and animals do not have Holy Spirit healing power.

Continuing to expose this intertwined healing method, we find a mixture of spiritual passions that are not Biblical.

> By means of the Reiki power, we have the possibility of uniting heaven and earth.... The theoretical roots of Reiki are found in a colorful mixture of Mikkyo Buddhism, Chinese Qigong, and Japanese Shintoism.[9]

By the time you have finished reading all of the Reiki information that is presented, it will be obvious the United States of America has embraced a type of healing energy that is not from the Holy Spirit and was not used by Jesus or His disciples. In fact, the reception of Reiki healing energy is sweeping the continents of the world.

Mikao Usui, the Student

Usui's interests ranged from biographies, history, medicine, psychology and theology (including Buddhist and Christian) to astrology, incantations (such as removing sickness), physiognomy (face reading) shinsen no jitsu (God hermit technique) and divination. (https://reikiinmedicine.org/popular/mikao-usui-reiki-healing/)

Insight: The wide range of Dr. Usui's interests shows he had significant exposure to occult practices. Such exposure can allow evil spirits into one's presence.

The Founder of Reiki

The history of Reiki begins with its founder, Dr. Mikao Usui. Sometimes called the Usui Sensei, Dr. Mikao was born to a wealthy Buddhist family…. As a child, Dr. Usui studied in a Buddhist monastery where he was taught martial arts, swordsmanship, and the Japanese form of Chi Kung, known as Kiko… It was his desire to find a method of healing that was unattached to any specific religion and religious belief, so that his system would be accessible to everyone.

Spiritual Awakening, Reiki Development

Sometime during his years of training in the monastery, Dr. Usui attended his own training rediscovery course in a cave on Mount Kurama. For 21 days, Dr. Usui fasted, meditated and prayed. On the morning of the twenty-first day, Dr. Usui experienced an event that would change his life forever. He saw ancient Sanskrit symbols that helped him develop the system of healing he had been struggling to invent. Usui Reiki was born. (https://iarp.org/history-of-reiki).

Insight: This was *not* an encounter with the healing power of Christ's Holy Spirit, because the Holy Spirit doesn't need to "develop" a system of healing derived from Sanskrit symbols. The fast Dr. Usui participated in is called "The Lotus Repentance," which comes from Tendai Buddhism. The change or enlightenment (satori) that Dr. Usui experienced led to his reception of the Reiki healing energy. Mount Kurama has been described as being "the spiritual heart of Japan," a place with many temples representing a whole range of deities. Deities are also called "gods," "spirits," and "demons."

Usui Sensei passed away in 1926, and in remembrance of him the Usui memorial was erected at the Saihoji Temple in Tokyo, Japan. There is a long inscription on the monument giving details about his life, his values, and the Reiki method he started. Nothing is mentioned in the inscription about him being a Christian, a devout follower of Jesus as the Savior,

Son of God, or proclaiming the Bible as the Word of God. (http://www.reiki.org/faq/HistoryOfReiki.html).

Insight: From the sources presented, it is obvious that Reiki healers do not use Holy Spirit power to heal as Jesus and His apostles did. You can call Reiki power "universal life energy," "God energy," "life force energy," "Radiance Technique Energy," "Prana," "Chi," "Ki," or whatever you want, but when compared to the Bible it is *not* the Holy Spirit power that comes from the Almighty God. For a better understanding about Reiki energy, some detailed information on "the source" of Reiki energy will now be revealed.

Reiki Energy - What is it? How does it heal?

The word Reiki is composed of two Japanese words – Rei and Ki. When translating Japanese into English, we must keep in mind that an exact translation is difficult. The Japanese language has many levels of meaning. Therefore, the context of the word being used must be kept in mind when attempting to communicate its essence. Because these words are being used in a spiritual healing context, a Japanese/English dictionary does not provide the depth of meaning we seek, as its definitions are based on common everyday Japanese. As an example, *Rei is often defined as ghost and Ki as vapor* and while these words vaguely point in the direction of meaning we seek, they fall far short of the understanding that is needed. (My emphasis).

When seeking a definition from a more spiritual context, we find that Rei can be defined as the Higher Intelligence that guides the creation and functioning of the universe. Rei is a subtle wisdom that permeates everything, both animate and inanimate…. Because of its infinite nature, it is all knowing. Rei is also called God and has many other names depending on the culture that has named it.

Ki is the non-physical energy that animates all living things. Ki is flowing in everything that is alive, including plants, animals and humans. (My comment: Bible proof of Ki in all humans?). (http://www.reiki.org/reikinews/whatislg.html).

Insight: Rei (ghost) Ki (vapor), in describing this healing technique, verifies it is linked with occult healing where ghosts (evil spirits) are found. If the ghost vapor of Reiki healing was truly the Holy Ghost from the LORD, He would glorify Jesus and testify about Him (John 15:26). And if Rei is a Higher Intelligence, also called God, who guides creation and the functioning of the universe, then this would indicate that Rei is God almighty, which is not true, because God the Father was and is revealed through Jesus (John 14:6-9). Rei is also referred to as all-knowing and infinite, attributes that alone belong to the LORD God of the Bible. If Reiki has intelligence, then this energy force qualifies as an intelligent spiritual power that counterfeits the nature and healing power of the true God and His Holy Spirit. No one who claims to be a Christian should be using or receiving Reiki healing or any therapy linked to Reiki.

Alarming Information on Reiki Power

Several website sources giving details about Reiki will now be presented so that you will have no doubt as to what constitutes Reiki healing.

Reiki Energy develops your aura, chakras and your meridians…. The Reiki Energy is a specific form of "hands on" energy healing developed in Japan. A Reiki Energy practitioner channels energy from the infinite reservoir around himself and directs it into the recipient's energy field. (Page 1).

An attunement is an energetic connection that is passed on from the Reiki practitioner to the student. It will open up channels to the receiver to allow them to access the particular Reiki modality that the person is attuned to. There are other names for an attunement, like empowerment…. Typically when an energy system is formed, it is either channeled by one or several practitioners and they first receive an attunement from Spirit, or the Ascended Master, Archangel, Fairies, etc., and are gifted with the knowledge on how to attune and share that energy with others. (Page 2). (http://www.spiritualhealing-now.com/reiki-energy.html).

Insight: Anyone with basic occult knowledge knows that aura reading, the seven chakras, *and* meridians all have a direct link with witchcraft. So if Reiki energy develops these systems, then it develops your channeled connection to demons, because demons abound in all areas of the occult. The laying on of hands to any body part establishes a "contact point" and is common in universal energy healing. Contact points also allow available demonic energy to be channeled or transferred from one person to another. The word "attunement" implies that one is choosing to come into agreement, harmony, or accord with what is being offered. In this case, the attunement is accepting the power and influence from a power of something other than the Holy Spirit. Names or titles of healing power sources such as Archangel, Fairies, Spirit, and Ascended Master are found in New Age and occult teachings. There is only one true Spirit, the Holy Spirit Jesus talked about in John, chapters 14-16. And there is only one true Ascended Master! The true Ascended Master is the resurrected Lord Jesus, Who ascended to heaven after He was raised from the dead (Luke 24:5-7; Acts 1:9-11; 1 Corinthians 15:3-8).

Universal Energy takes everything you say quite literally…. Some people learn how to use this Energy through the study and practice of Wicca or other forms of Witchcraft and real magic. Others learn by practicing yoga or meditation. (http://www.mistressofmagic.com/article/spiritualenergy.html).

Insight: This short piece of information shows clearly that Universal Energy, the same energy used in Reiki healing, is available in witchcraft. The Holy Spirit is *not* available in Wicca healing or any form of witchcraft healing. If this Universal Energy can take (understand) literally what we say, that means this energy has intelligence capable of changing a sound mind to embrace evil and deceptive teachings.

Welcome to Magic Touch and Energy Work. I am a certified Reiki Grand Master and Integrated Energy Therapy Practitioner. I use intuition and angel guidance to heal each client. I also use pendulums and crystals if guided to do so. I can clear and balance chakras and can communicate with your higher self to heal you…. I also use pendulums and my guides to dowse for water and find lost objects. (http://magictouchhealing.com/index.html).

Insight: Here we find a certified Reiki Grand Master who uses angel guidance and objects for Reiki energy healing. Pendulums, guides, and crystals are also used to accomplish healing, to help find lost objects, and locate water. The Jesus of the Bible did not use pendulums, crystals, angels, or spirit guides to heal people, nor did He clear and balance chakras. His healings were done by the power of the Holy Spirit, according to the will of His Father. And the followers of Jesus, who were given supernatural power to heal, healed *only* by the power of the Holy Spirit in the Name of Jesus (Acts 3:1-9; 5:14-16; 9:33-35; 28:8-9). God's gift of healing is only from Holy Spirit power (1 Corinthians 12:9, 11), not from any other spiritual energy source.

A Reiki Healing Affirmation:

An Affirmation: I invoke the Healing Buddha and the Master Spirits of Reiki. I ask that my channel be pure and clean, without fear, and with honor and love for all. (Page 4). (http://reiki.7gen.com/).

Insight: This four page article talks about Reiki's capabilities and finishes with this prayer (affirmation) to the healing Buddha and Master Reiki spirits. So where did Buddha get his healing power, if he had any? If it was not from Jesus, then it must have been from the occult where evil healing spirits reside, longing to counterfeit the Holy Spirit healings.

There are Reiki symbols (special signs and hieroglyphs) that are used to speed up the process of connecting a person to high energies during Reiki degree initiation or attunement. The use of these Reiki symbols does not require meditation or many years of spiritual practices. That is what many Reiki masters and teachers of Karuna, Usui, and Kundalini schools allegedly affirm. These Reiki symbols influence the subconscious mind, change the inner state of a person and give the ability to connect to a higher spiritual energy source. (http://www.lifexpert.com/special/reiki.html).

Insight: What is it about Reiki symbols that speed up the process of connecting a person to "high energies" during Reiki degree initiation or attunement? In witchcraft, symbols are used to attract or make demons feel welcome. Could these Japanese symbols be "contact points" for evil spirits to hang around in order to influence the subconscious mind of a new Reiki initiate, and also change the inner state of a person? In my personal and direct experience in casting demons out of people, I can tell you that when a demon (evil spirit) enters or leaves a person, the inner state of the person is changed. If the Reiki symbols truly give a person the ability to connect to a higher "spiritual energy source" and it is not the Holy Spirit, then most likely it is an evil spiritual energy force that opposes the Holy Spirit healing of Almighty God.

…The ability to do Reiki healing is simply channeled through the Reiki master to the practitioner during the attunement process. Years of study and discipline are not necessary. Imagine my surprise during my first Reiki class when I observed the astral images of guides and healing spirits pouring forth bright shimmering rays of healing energy at the hands of novice practitioners only three hours after the class first started! (My comment: Is this an occult loaded energy class?). (http://reiki.org/reikinews/reikin19.html).

Insight: This Reiki participant observed "astral images of guides and healing spirits" that poured "forth bright shimmering rays of healing energy" through the hands of novice Reiki practitioners *only* three hours after the class had started. Such eye witness information should send a clear and alarming message to all who want no contact with evil spirits. The Reiki supernatural energy healing power described in the above quote establishes the fact that "guides" (occult term for spirits) and healing spirits (more than one spirit) were seen at this first Reiki setting. The channeled healing energy from this attunement matches the description of what some call "spiritual energy transference." This type of spiritual energy is capable of transferring an evil spirit into a person. In the Bible, the Holy Spirit is the *only* Spirit that does God's healing. In our diverse world of various energy beliefs and witchcraft healing practices, evil spirits can masquerade as healing energy to do the healing.

Reiki is promoted/advertised as a safe and gentle form of hands-on healing. Reiki initiation attunes a practitioner to become a channel for the Reiki energy and to provide life-changing experiences for physical, mental, and spiritual growth. The training can include the history, scientific evidence of Reiki energy, how to prepare a room for Reiki, and the various techniques for performing Reiki treatments. Normally, there are three levels of learning in order to advance one's Reiki healing power.

- Level I Reiki connects the practitioner to the Reiki energy and teaches hands-on Reiki
- Level II Reiki teaches the practitioner long distance or remote healing
- Level III Reiki initiates the practitioner to become a Reiki Master

Each level has its own set of attunements and techniques for the type of Reiki to be practiced. Once a person has received these attunements, they are Reiki practitioners capable of channeling the Reiki energy. Reiki initiations are for life. Fees and lengths of teaching time vary for Reiki classes with different Reiki Masters.

Some Reiki masters offer Level I, II, and III in a single weekend. Most prefer to do each level separately, because some Reiki students report the attunements cause changes in all aspects of their lives to which the practitioner needs time to adjust. Because of this, most Reiki Masters do not combine Level I, II, and III classes. They allow practitioners time to adjust and gain the benefits of each attunement.

Insight: These three levels, sometimes called sessions of attunement, are mentioned for Reiki initiation (some Reiki Masters teach more than three levels). Each session takes the initiate deeper into the Reiki realm of supernatural energy power. Level II teaches that a Reiki practitioner can do long distance healing. How can this be if Reiki is *only* spiritual energy? There must be intelligence in the Reiki energy if it can be sent long distance and accomplish a specific purpose. So what or who is this intelligence, if it is not the Holy Spirit? Could it be that *the other* intelligent healing power is found in the occult where evil spirits dwell? A former witch, who became a Christian, told me her ability to heal while active in healing came from a demonic healing spirit that was not from God. Demonic healing is common in witchcraft. Holy Spirit healing comes from the Lord God. It is not done by levels of attunement, nor is God's healing energy circulating the world for any to use at will. If Reiki energy is from God and *anyone* can use it, then God can be *forced* to heal those who hate Him, curse Him, curse His Son, deny His eternal existence, trash the Bible, and refuse to accept the forgiveness of all their sins through faith in Jesus Christ. Such a belief is blasphemy and bypasses the Name of Jesus (1 John 5:13-14) and God's will in healing (1 Corinthians 12:9, 11).

I have a good friend of more than thirty years. He was born into a Hawaiian bloodline that has practiced Kahuna witchcraft for over three hundred years. He renounced it and became a Christian. I watched as he had various demonic spirits cast out of him. He had been given occult healing power from a specific indwelling demon. He told me a story about his aunt who lived in Hawaii and still practiced Kahuna witchcraft. She heard her nephew in Oregon had broken his forearm. It had been in a cast less than two weeks when she heard of this. She phoned her nephew and told him to go to the doctor for an x-ray to prove it was healed and no longer needed a cast. The boy went to the doctor. An x-ray confirmed that it was completely healed. He should have been in a cast for six weeks.

She sent a demonic spirit from Hawaii to Oregon to heal her nephew and the demon did it in one visit. This is "distance healing," exactly what is taught and being done in Reiki healing and other types of energy healing classes. Are you now seeing the unholy foundation of Reiki energy? Do you need to repent and get out of it? Only the Lord Jesus has the power to cancel your Reiki initiation, forgive your sins (Acts 4:12), and protect you from this deceptive evil way of healing that is *not* from His Holy Spirit.

Two pages earlier, Reiki's three levels of attunements were "bullet" explained. They are done separately because "the attunements cause changes in all aspects of their lives to which the practitioners need time to adjust." Spiritual energy that can change all aspects in a person's life must be "intelligent and powerful." Demons have intelligence and power, and I have seen demons slowly or quickly change a person's life for evil, rather than good. If the spiritual change does not lead to seeking Jesus for repentance of sins, and demons don't teach repentance in the Name of Jesus, then the spiritual change is *against* the Lord Jesus and His Holy Spirit.

Reiki initiates pay money to receive attunements for Reiki healing power. Jesus freely gave His apostles authority to heal as recorded in Matthew 10:1 and Luke 9:1-2. He did not charge them any money or require for them to go through levels of attunements to receive the ability to heal people. This true gift of healing was and is bestowed upon specific people according to the will of Almighty God. According to Biblical teaching, Reiki healing power is not from the God Who created heaven and earth and forgives your sins.

Reiki Treatments Are Common in Hospitals

During my search for Reiki information I was surprised to find out how common and wide spread Reiki healing is among hospitals in America and throughout the world. The pieces of information that will follow should convince you that "the evil spiritual energy healing realm" is big and acceptable in many hospitals and medical centers.

Today there is a steady increase of holistic health practices being integrated into the allopathic community. In recent years the popularity of Reiki healing, a Japanese method of natural healing, appears to have taken a forefront in many mainstream areas. Clearly Energy Healing and Energy Medicine are becoming an accepted and sought after practice in medical clinics, the doctor's office, and hospitals throughout the world. Reiki is simply a natural progression in the exponential growth of healthcare services today. A subtitle on this webpage is called **The Spirit of our Program** and it boldly proclaims: "We intend to expand our presence and contribution as a recognizable complement to the existing quality care already present as it perpetuates the credibility and value of Reiki in the hospital environment." (http://hospitalreiki.com/index.htm).

Insight: The above paragraph shows how Reiki is "becoming an accepted and sought after practice" in various medical fields and "is simply a natural progression in the exponential growth of healthcare services today." They are determined ("We intend") to expand their presence and credibility and the value of Reiki in the hospital environment. Truly, prayer for protection from evil energy activity is a must when going to *any* medical facility. Find out information about doctors and medical facilities before you commit your money and offer your body for any type of treatment. Christians, your body is the temple of the Holy Spirit (1 Corinthians 6:19). God does not want you to receive energy healing from an unholy universal spiritual source at any time. Seek the Lord Jesus for any needed healing (1 Corinthians 12:9, 11) and have Christians fast and pray for you.

The Center for Reiki Research Including Reiki in Hospitals

Reiki is a method of stress reduction that promotes healing. It is ministered by laying-on hands. Lay practitioners have used it for more than 90 years, and its popularity is growing. A study done in 2007 by the National Health Interview Survey indicates that 1.2 million adults and 161,000 children received one or more sessions of energy healing therapy such as Reiki in the previous year. According to the American Hospital Association, in 2007, 15% or over 800 American hospitals offered Reiki as part of hospital services. (http://www.centerforreikiresearch.org/).

Insight: This 2007 study shows clearly that Reiki healing/therapy has made extensive progress in penetrating the medical field and involving multitudes with "another healing power," one not from the Lord Jesus. As I type this in 2018, it would seem reasonable to say the numbers involved with Reiki have risen. It is shocking to know children are being directly exposed to Reiki. One can only wonder how many Reiki ignorant adults are exposing their children to an anti-Holy Spirit energy force that will fight against them when they hear the Gospel about Jesus and His forgiveness. Could this "energy force" be the source of teen rebellion in some households and schools? The spiritual implications could bring eternal consequences. Parents are to be spiritual guardians of their children. Matthew 18:5-6 says they will be held accountable if they mislead their children.

The International Center for Reiki Training

At hospitals and clinics across America, Reiki is beginning to gain acceptance as a meaningful and cost-effective way to improve patient care…. "Reiki sessions cause people to heal faster with less pain," says Marilyn Vega, RN, a private duty nurse at the Manhattan Eye, Ear and Throat Hospital in New York…. Vega, a Reiki master, includes Reiki with her regular nursing procedures…. Patients have asked her to do Reiki on them in the operating and recovery rooms…. Reiki was in use in hospital operating rooms as early as the mid-90's. Since then its acceptance in medicine has grown. It is now listed in a nursing "scope and standards of practice" publication as an accepted form of care. (Page 1). (http://www.reiki.org/reikinews/reiki_in_hospitals.html).

Insight: This article is titled ***Reiki In Hospitals*** by William Lee Rand. The information establishes the fact that Reiki has been used in hospitals as early as the mid-90's, and it continues to gain acceptance as an important healing therapy. Reiki spiritual energy does have the ability to heal in some cases and that's why some think it is "good healing energy." This is what makes this energy healing therapy seem okay or harmless, because it does bring comfort at times. I know a former demonic healer who later became a Christian. She had the ability to heal and saw miraculous occult healings. One healing was third degree burned tissue in the palm of a car mechanic, which was restored in less than a minute. The other was the spine of a hunchback that flattened and straightened out within a minute. There was no pain or unpleasant presence during these healings, only relief from the problem. For evil spirit healing to deceive people, the spirits must induce some type of warm or relaxing feeling to the willing recipient.

How Does Reiki Heal?

All forms of healing whether traditional, complimentary, or alternative have an impact on the human subtle energy system. Each method also carries a unique vibrational frequency and consequently will create different effects…. Reiki is being embraced by many prestigious hospitals where it is offered as a part of standard care.

…Reiki…may ultimately be the most important alternative treatment of all… (My comment: Jesus is the true healer). (http://www.reikiclasses.com/reikiclasses/?p=30).

Insight: To say that each healing method has its own "unique vibrational frequency" means there are different types of energy matter around us. So does each form of healing have its own specific "spiritual" energy matter? Or would it be more accurate to believe there are numerous evil spirits with different attunement levels and varieties of deceptive healing powers that are luring people into their evil healing realm? These website comments about Reiki once again show the strong medical approval of a healing method that was not taught by the Lord Jesus, so it does not have the Lord's approval. Are you embracing healing methods not taught by

Jesus, the Son of God, the only Savior of the world from its sins (Acts 4:12)?

Ray Yungen has written a book called *For Many Shall Come in My Name* (Lighthouse Trails Publishing). Within pages 78-81, he documents some startling information about Reiki. On page 79 it reads: "Over *one million* people are practicing Reiki in the United States alone today. In many cases, these are people who treat or work with others on a therapeutic basis, such as health professionals, body workers, chiropractors, and counselors…. In Europe alone, the number of people accepting Reiki is very impressive. One Reiki master claims that in the thirteen years she lived in Europe she alone initiated 45,000 people into Reiki as channelers."

On page 80 of his book, a letter found in the *Reiki Journal* reveals: "Reiki is a whole new experience when used in my massage therapy practice. Massage, I thought, would be an excellent tool to spread the radiance of this universal energy and a client would benefit and really *not realize what a wonderful growth was happening in his or her being*" (Emphasis Ray Yungen). The fact that some do not realize energy transfer is occurring when receiving Reiki massage therapy should sound the alarm to all. There was nothing sneaky or devious about the Holy Spirit healings Jesus did. People knew exactly what was happening when He was healing people in public or private, as stated in the Gospels.

Since Reiki is not something taught intellectually, even children can be easily deceived into accepting it. Ray Yungen found an ad that offered a children's Reiki book called, *Children's Reiki Handbook: A Guide to Energy Healing for Kids*. The book is described as a "guide that provides kids with what they need to prepare for their first Reiki Attunement" (page 81). This sounds more like preparing a kid for the first step into the occult. Any initiation, ritual, or attunement to receive a supernatural spiritual energy transfer is transferring the safety of one's soul *away* from the love and protection of Jesus Christ.

The previous six pages showed the devastating penetration of Reiki into various medical fields and into the lives of young children. When permitted and not resisted, evil sets no boundaries. Whenever you have surgery or any medical treatment at a hospital, remember to tell the people working with you that you do not want any help from Reiki medical treatments or any type of energy healing therapy, and pray for protection from any distance energy healing. The next two sub-headings will disclose what the Reiki symbols represent.

What the Reiki Healing Symbols Represent

Some Reiki masters display the Reiki symbols, while others keep them hidden and expose them only to the new initiates during their attunements. During my research on these symbols, I found them at various websites. I will display only the main Reiki symbol. As the definitions of other symbols are presented, you will see a progression of intended spiritual guidance which takes the initiate deeper into the Reiki realm in order to achieve a variety of energy healing abilities.

The Japanese Character of Reiki

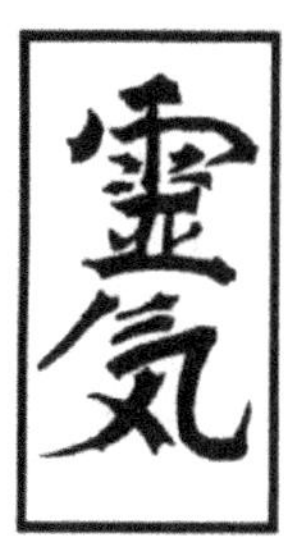

If you see this symbol in a home, medical facility, doctor's office, chiropractor's office, or physical therapy center, you are in a place that welcomes and uses occult Reiki energy for various types of healings. Find other medical help where this symbol is not advertised. Find a place where the best medical treatment is available and where prayer in the Name of Jesus is given. Next, the meaning of basic Reiki symbols.

Reiki Symbols are means of focusing your attention in order to connect with "specific" healing frequencies. Using different symbols will boost up the Reiki energy. (Page 1).

Meaning of Reiki symbols:

CHO KU RAY

Pronunciation choh-koo-ray

Alias: The **Power** Symbol

67

Meaning: "God and Man Coming Together" or "I have the key." The primary use of this Symbol is to increase Reiki power. It draws Energy from around you and it focuses it where you want to… It is the all-purpose symbol. It can be used for anything, anywhere… on food, water, medicine, herbs, cleaning negative energies, spiritual protection, in sick rooms and hospitals, to aid manifestation, to empower other Reiki Symbols, and to seal energies after treatment. (Page 2).

SEI HEI KI

Pronunciation: say-hay-key

Alias: The **Mental/Emotional** Symbol

Meaning: "God and Man Coming Together" or "Key to the Universe." It is used primarily for mental/emotional healing and calming the mind. It is very good for: psychic protection, cleansing, in meditations to activate Kundalini energy, to balance the left and right brain, aid for removing addictions, for healing past traumas, clearing emotional blockages, aligning the upper chakras, removing negative energies and bad vibrations and restores emotional balance and harmony. (Pages 2, 3).

HON SHA ZE SHO NEN

Pronunciation: hanh-shah-zay-show-nen

Alias: The **Distance** Symbol

Meaning: "The God (The Buddha, the Christ…) in Me Greets the God in You to Promote Enlightenment and Peace." This is the Distance Healing Symbol and it is used to send Reiki over distance and time (past, present, future), to anyone and anything. It is also drawn when sending a distant attunement. (Page 3).

TAM-A-RA-SHA

Pronunciation: tam-ara-sha

Alias: The **Balancing** Factor

It is a balancing/unblocking Symbol. It grounds and balances energy, helps to unblock the energy chakra centers, allowing the energy to flow, and helps to reduce and dissipate pain. (Page 4).

THE REIKI MASTER SYMBOL

DAI KO MYO

Pronunciation: dye-ko-me-o

Alias: The **Master** Symbol

It is the most powerful symbol in the Reiki group. It can be used only by Reiki Masters. This symbol is used to heal the soul. Since it deals with our soul and our spiritual self it heals disease and illness from the original source in the aura/energy fields. It helps to provide enlightenment and peace. It also allows to become more intuitive and psychic. (Pages 4-5). (http://www.reiki-for-holistichealth.com/reikisymbols.html).

 Insight: When one reads about the Reiki symbols just presented, it is obvious that they do not have a Holy Spirit connection. Any teaching incorporating symbols or objects for increasing spiritual power that promotes energy or chakra flows, and endorses meditations to activate Kundalini energy (known as serpent power) is teaching people to tune into *evil* spiritual frequencies. All of the miraculous Holy Spirit healings demonstrated by Jesus and His apostles never needed any symbols for healing, because the true God does not need "symbol" help when providing His spiritual and physical healing power.

Reiki's Direct Connection with Witchcraft

This final section of information on the power source of Reiki energy will show that it is a form of Spiritism (contacting the dead who supposedly have ascended to a higher level). This spiritual practice is found in witchcraft and forbidden in the Bible (Deuteronomy 18:9-12).

An article from **Reiki 101: Healing Energy Symbols and Spirit Guides:**

Part of Reiki includes the use of sacred symbols…. In addition to the symbols, however, *a Reiki practitioner may call upon spirit guides,* ascended masters, or angels depending on the spiritual path…. The practitioner focuses on the recipient's *chakra systems.* (My emphasis). (http://paganwiccan.about.com/od/dreamsandmeditation/p/R eiki_Intro.htm).

Insight: Calling upon spirit guides (demons) and ascended masters (people who have died) to send their spiritual energy into the chakra system is an ancient occult practice called "Spiritism" and has been used by witches for thousands of years. Focusing on the recipient's chakra system proves Reiki healing has no Holy Spirit healing connection.

The Llewellen Journal - Using Reiki Magick

As a practicing witch I use healing magick in my life all the time…. I know quite a few witches who get initiated into Reiki to supplement their magickal energy. *These witches use Reiki not just for healing, but also for many purposes.* They use Reiki energy to change candle spells, to consecrate herbal potions, and to cast the magick circle. (My emphasis). (http://www.llewellyn.com/journal/article/751).

Insight: From a practicing witch, we are told Reiki energy is compatible with magickal witchcraft energy when used "for healing" and "many purposes." Demonic spirits are involved with witchcraft healing, and Reiki energy supplements the demonic healings. This means demons and Reiki energy get along with each other and work together to heal. Since demons are evil and Reiki energy is welcomed to supplement various witchcraft purposes, then Reiki must be an evil force containing deceptive intelligence. Thus, Reiki is more than energy. It is a spiritual source of energy with intelligence for healing and its intelligence works with evil spirits, not the Holy Spirit. This proves Reiki is evil. The Holy Spirit will not allow demons to supplement His healing power.

One final piece of evidence should cement the fact that Reiki has a solid occult connection with the chakras. This web page information describes how Reiki works with the seven chakras or energy centers that some believe are found seated inside a person.

Reiki Chakras: The Energy Centers

In Reiki there are seven chakras or energy centers seated inside a person. (Page 1). In detailing chakra functions the article concludes by saying: These are the chakras that play a very crucial role in Reiki and in almost all of the traditional healing arts. (Page 4). (http://www.trainingreiki.com/reiki-chakras.php).

Insight: Chakra energy healing is commonly used in occult healings, can be found at various online websites, and in witchcraft books. Reiki healing energy travels through the seven chakras to produce healing and wellness. According to what the Bible teaches about Holy Spirit healing, there is no way Reiki healing power qualifies as being sent from the true God in heaven. Chakra healing was not taught or endorsed by Jesus. So who provides the power for Reiki healing? Think back on *all the detailed information* provided *from* Reiki websites. When compared to the Bible, do you now see and accept that the healing source for Reiki energy is *not* Holy Spirit energy, but unholy spiritual energy from evil spirits?

Those who claim to be Christians must renounce any and all involvement with Reiki healing or any energy healing, because it is not from the Lord Jesus. Symbols and all literature must be destroyed as directed from Acts 19:19-20. It is the evil one who seeks to devour (1 Peter 5:8) any who will fall for this deception. The LORD's Holy Spirit does not need help from the many Reiki evil spirits (guides) or "universal energy" when it comes to miraculous healings.

With all the evil information that has been provided on Reiki's origin and power to heal, why is it growing in acceptance worldwide? It is popular because most people who experience Reiki energy, but not all, say it is a pleasurable experience. They report a sense of warmth, being relaxed, and some report physical healing. Another reason Reiki is gaining global acceptance is that few people know about the information you have just read.

Just because something feels good doesn't mean it's from the true God. Ask former drug addicts how good they felt when on their drug of choice. When they were set free from the power of the drug that controlled their life, they realized how an evil drug made them feel good physically, emotionally, and mentally, but was leading them to a life of deception and possibly death. Has Reiki deceived you or some of your friends? The information being provided in this book needs to be shared with others for their protection.

Proponents of Reiki have referred to it as "a form of Divine Love" or "Limitless Love." However, there is no evidence in the Bible or in early Christian Church history that the followers of Jesus embraced and taught Reiki healing, any type of energy healing, or universal healing. Nor did they use symbols and attunements to get the LORD's Holy Spirit power. Reiki power is found in the occult where witchcraft is practiced. This was sufficiently documented for you. So if you really are a Christian, then the Holy Spirit should be the *only* Spirit you allow into your life for any type of comfort (John 15:26-27), strengthening, or healing.

Now that you know the truth, will you abide in the Lord Jesus so you can be free from deception and sin in this area? (John 8:31-32; 15:1-11). If you *are not* a Christian, please renounce the sin of Reiki involvement and *call upon the Lord Jesus to be forgiven, and saved from your sins* (Romans 10:9-13). Repent (confess it as sin) of any Reiki exposure or treatments you have undergone and dispose of all Reiki magazines and related objects.

If you are a Christian who has been involved with Reiki, you also need to repent of your Reiki sin involvement and dispose of all Reiki items. If your friends are in Reiki and won't repent of this sin, they are not servants and friends of Jesus Christ. So find some friends who will honor Jesus, the One with the *only* true Holy Spirit healing power.

The title on the cover "asked a question" as to whether Yoga and Reiki healing are evil. It's obvious. The multiple, detailed website facts provided have established the true answer. According to the Bible, both of these activities are evil and are not pleasing to God. Will you warn your friends?

All of humanity will one day stand before the judgement seat of the LORD (Romans 14:10; 2 Corinthians 5:10; Revelation 20:11-15). Establish your trust in the Lord Jesus (Proverbs 3:5-7) for healing your heart (Luke 4:18) and leading you to a personal and blessed relationship of love and forgiveness with His heavenly Father (John 1:12; 5:22-29; 14:6; Romans 10:9-13). Will I see you in heaven?

Resources used in this section:

1. Frank Arjava Petter, *Reiki The Legacy of Dr. Usui* (Twin Lakes, WI: Lotus Light Productions, 1998), p. 26.
2. Ibid., p. 27.
3. Dr. Mikao Usui and Frank Arjava Petter, *The Original Handbook of Dr. Mikao Usui* (Twin Lakes, WI: Lotus Press, 2011), p. 10.
4. Ibid., p. 4.
5. Frank Petter, *Reiki The Legacy of Dr. Usui*, pp. 28, 29.
6. Ibid., p. 9.
7. Ibid., p. 13.
8. Ibid., p. 19.
9. Ibid., p. 10.
10. Ray Yungen, *For Many Shall Come in My Name* (Silverton, Oregon: Lighthouse Trails Publishing, 2007), pp. 78-81.